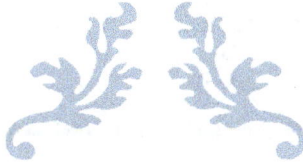

Type 2 Diabetes Recipes

Your All-Purpose Guide To Easy, Healthy And Delicious Recipes
For Type 2 Diabetes And Whole Health With Simple And Healthy
Diabetic Recipes To Manage Diabetes And Prediabetes

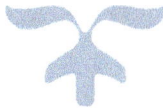

Isabella Miller

the author is not engaging in the rendering of legal, financial, medical or professional advice. The content within this book has been derived from various sources. Please consult a licensed professional before attempting any techniques outlined in this book.

By reading this document, the reader agrees that under no circumstances is the author responsible for any losses, direct or indirect, which are incurred as a result of the use of information contained within this document, including, but not limited to, errors, omissions, or inaccuracies.

Table of Contents

Breakfast and Brunch

1. Strawberry Banana Smoothie
Preparation Time: 4 Minutes
Cooking Time: 0 minutes
Servings: 2
Total budget: 5$
Ingredients
- 1 handful chia seeds
- 1 cup strawberries, hulled
- 1 cup bananas, sliced
- 1 cup milk
- 1 handful ice cubes

Directions
Mix the 5 ingredients in a food processor. Blend till you get a fine and smooth mixture.

Nutrition
Calories: 37 kcal   **Total Fat:** 0 g   **Protein:** 13 g

2. Cinnamon Pumpkin Waffles

Preparation Time: 15 minutes
Cooking Time: 5 minutes per waffle
Servings: 2
Total budget: 8$

Ingredients

- 1 cup buttermilk
- 1 large egg
- ¼ cup pumpkin, canned
- ¾ tsp. ground cinnamon
- 1 tsp. molasses
- 2 tsps. canola oil
- ⅛ tsp. ground nutmeg
- ½ tsp. ground ginger
- ½ tsp. baking soda
- ¼ tsp. sea salt
- 1 tsp. baking powder
- 1 cup all-purpose flour
- 1 ½ cups sugar-free maple syrup
- 2 tbsps. Splenda

Directions

Preheat waffle iron according to the manufacturer's directions, then spray lightly with cooking spray.

Mix baking powder, flour, baking soda, ginger, salt, cinnamon, and nutmeg in a large mixing bowl and set aside. Mix the molasses, pumpkin, oil, and buttermilk in another bowl, then set aside.

Whisk your egg and Splenda until well combined. Add the buttermilk mixture, continue to whisk to blend. Add the dry ingredients and stir. Pour the batter into hot waffle iron and bake for about 5 minutes. Serve with sugar-free maple syrup.

Nutrition
Calories: 160 kcal   **Total Fat:** 3 g   **Protein:** 5 g

3. Banana Pancakes
Preparation Time: 5 minutes
Cooking Time: 1 minute per side
Serving: 2
Total budget: 9$

Ingredients
- 2 ripe bananas, peeled
- 1 tsp. vanilla extract
- 3 eggs
- 1 tsp. baking powder
- ¼ tsp. cinnamon

Directions
In a mixing bowl, mash your bananas until mushy. Add the remaining ingredients and whisk until well combined. Coat your skillet or griddle with some cooking spray and heat over medium-high heat until hot. Add ⅛ of a cup batter for each pancake onto the griddle and cook for about 1-2 minutes per side. Continue to cook until batter is used.

Nutrition
Calories: 37 kcal   **Total Fat:** 1 g   **Protein:** 2 g

4. Pumpkin Walnut Oatmeal
Preparation Time: 5 minutes
Cooking Time: 5 minutes
Servings: 2
Total budget: 9$
Ingredients

- 1 cup soy milk
- ½ cup oats, old-fashioned and rolled
- ¼ cup pumpkin puree, canned
- 1 tbsp. walnuts, chopped
- 3 dashes ground cinnamon
- ½ tsp. honey

Directions

Mix the soy milk, oats, pumpkin puree, and cinnamon in a pan. Bring your mixture to a gentle boil, then reduce heat to low and simmer for 5 minutes. Add mixture to a serving bowl and garnish with walnuts and honey. Serve and enjoy!

Nutrition

Calories: 244 kcal **Total Fat:** 10 g **Protein:** 10.9 g

Lunch Vegetable Recipes

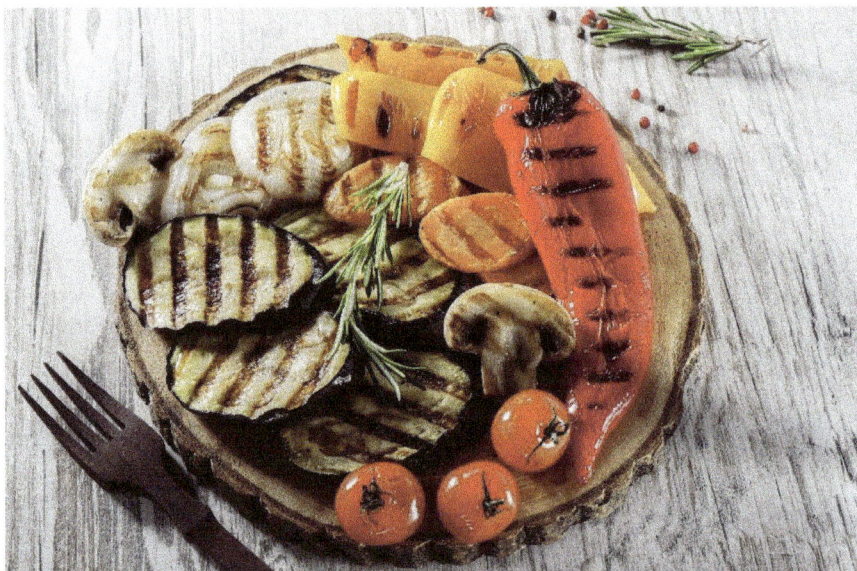

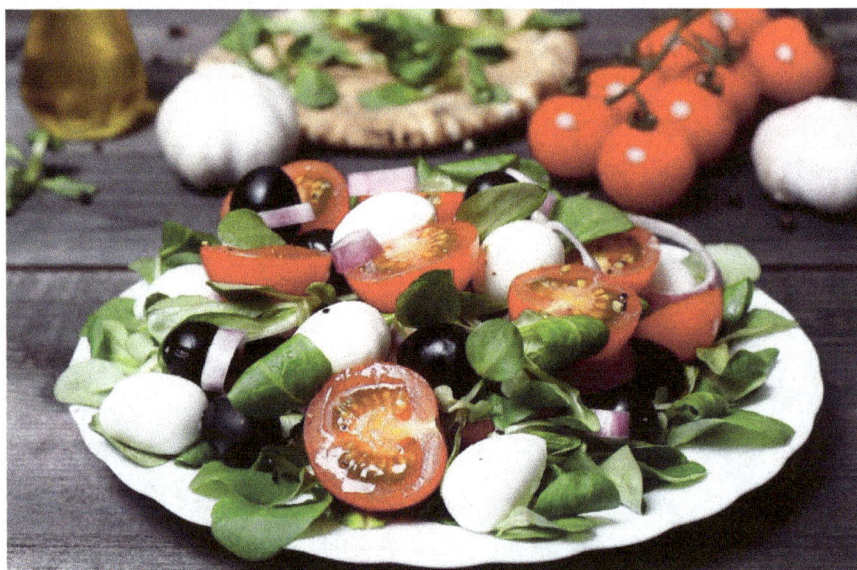

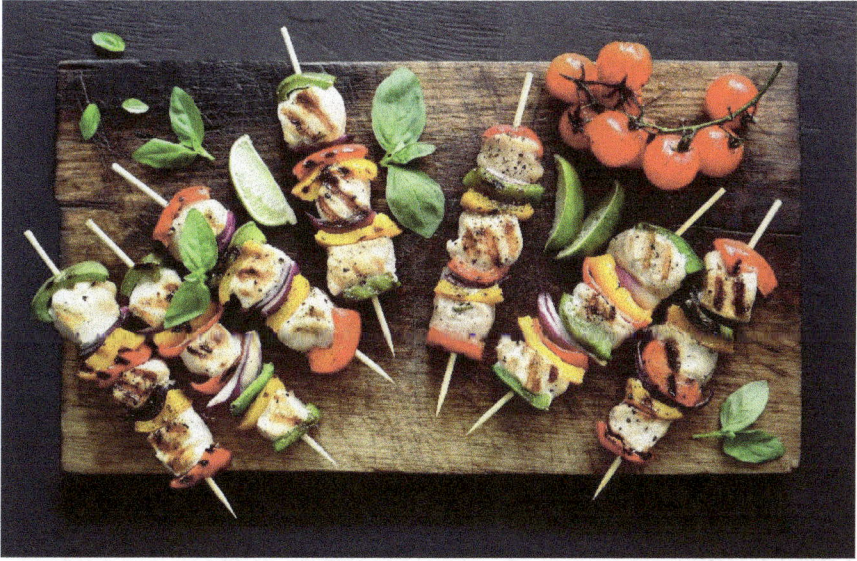

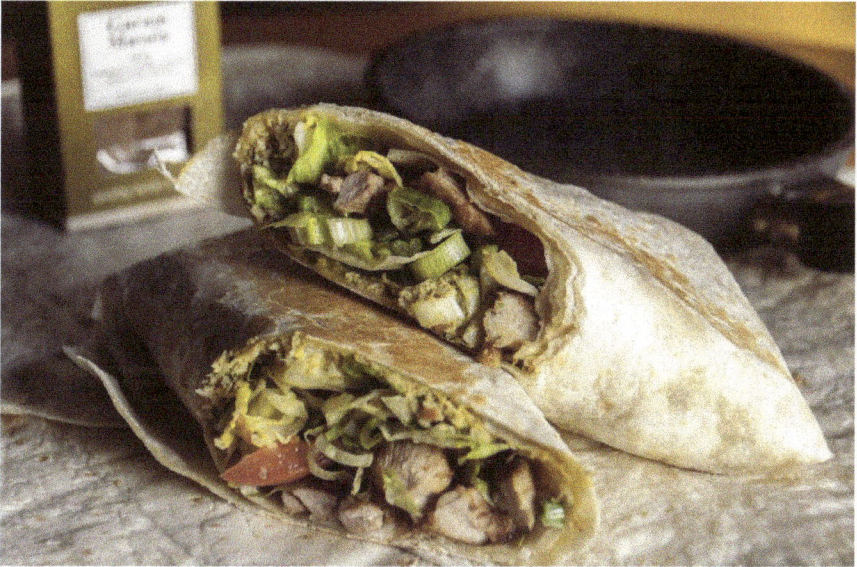

1. Balsamic-Roasted Broccoli

Preparation Time: 10 min
Cooking Time: 15 min
Servings: 2
Total budget: 16$

Ingredients

- 1 lb. broccoli
- 1 tbsp. extra virgin olive oil
- 1 tbsp. balsamic vinegar
- 1 clove garlic
- ⅛ tsp. salt
- Pepper to taste

Directions

Preheat oven to 450°F. Combine broccoli, olive oil, vinegar, minced garlic, salt, and pepper, toss. Spread broccoli on a baking sheet. Bake 12 to 15 min.

Nutrition

Calories: 27 kcal **Total Fat:** 0.3 g **Protein:** 3 g

2. Cauliflower Muffin
Preparation Time: 10 min
Cooking Time: 15 min
 Servings: 2
Total budget: 15$
Ingredients

- 2 ½ cup cauliflower
- ⅔ cup ham
- 2 ½ cups cheese
- ⅔ cup champignon
- 1 ½ tbsps. flaxseed
- 3 eggs
- ¼ tsp. salt
- ⅛ tsp. pepper

Directions

Preheat oven to 375°F. Put muffin liners in a 12-muffin tin. Combine cauliflower, ground flaxseed, beaten eggs, cup diced ham, grated cheese, diced mushrooms, salt, and pepper. Divide mixture rightly between muffin liners. Bake 30 minutes. This is a great lunch for the whole family.

Nutrition
Calories: 116 kcal   **Total Fat:** 7 g   **Protein:** 10 g

Lunch Meat Recipes

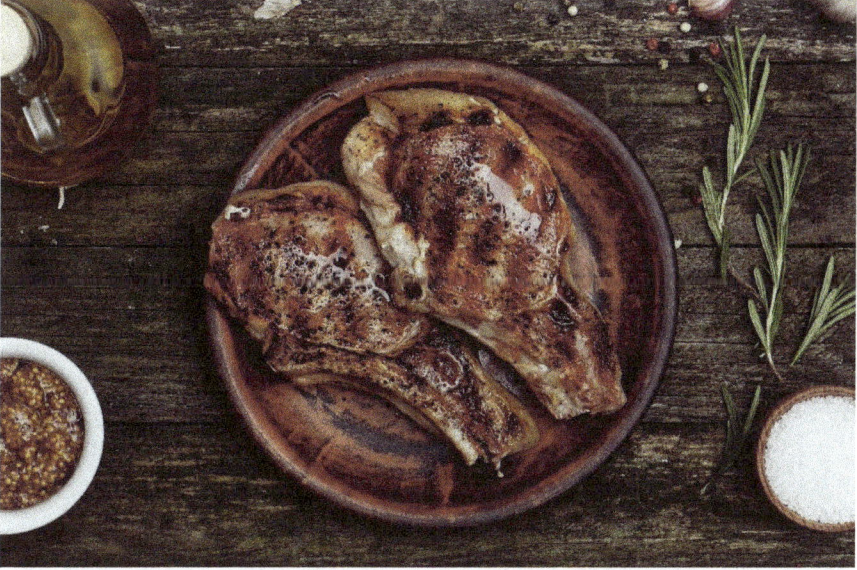

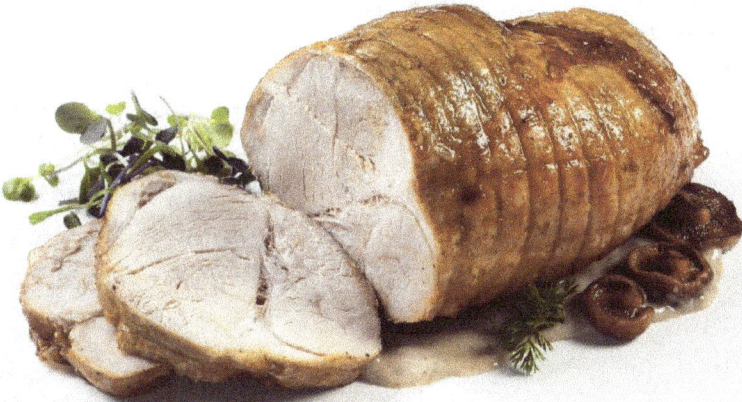

1. Spicy Brisket

Preparation Time: 5 minutes
Cooking Time: 110 minutes
Servings: 2
Total budget: 11$

Ingredients

- 3 tsps. salt
- 2 tsps. pepper
- 1 tsp. garlic powder
- 1 tsp. thyme, dried
- ½ tsp. rosemary, dried
- 1 (5-lb.) beef brisket
- 1 tsp. avocado oil
- 1 cup beef broth
- ½ cup jalapeno juice, pickled
- ½ cup jalapenos, pickled
- ½ onion, chopped

Directions

In a bowl, combine rosemary, thyme, garlic powder, pepper, and salt. Rub the brisket with the mixture and set aside. Warm the avocado oil over Sauté in the Instant Pot. Sear each side of the brisket for 5 minutes. Add onions, jalapenos, jalapeno juice, and broth to the Instant Pot. Close the lid and press Manual. Cook for 100 minutes. Do a natural release for 30 to 40 minutes. Avoid quick release. Remove the brisket, and slice. Pour with the strained broth and serve.

Nutrition

Calories: 101 kcal   **Total Fat:** 68.3 g   **Protein:** 62 g

2. Lime Pulled Pork

Preparation Time: 5 minutes
Cooking Time: 30 minutes
Servings: 2
Total budget: 11$

Ingredients

- 1 tbsp. Chili adobo sauce
- 1 tbsp. Chili powder
- 2 tsps. salt
- 1 tsp. garlic powder
- 1 tsp. cumin
- ½ tsp. pepper
- 2 ½ to 3 lb. pork, cubed
- 1 tbsp. coconut oil
- 2 cups beef broth
- 1 lime, cut into wedges
- ¼ cup cilantro, chopped

Directions

In a bowl, mix pepper, cumin, garlic powder, salt, chili powder, and sauce. Melt the oil on Sauté in the Instant Pot. Rub the pork with spice mixture. Place pork and sear for 3 to 5 min. per side.

Add broth and close the lid. Press Manual and cook 30 minutes. Do a natural release and open.

Shred pork. If you want crispy pork, then heat in a skillet until the pork is crisp. Serve warm with cilantro garnish and fresh lime wedges.

Nutrition

Calories: 570 kcal **Total Fat:** 35 g **Protein:** 55 g

3. Chipotle Pork Chops

Preparation Time: 7 minutes
Cooking Time: 15 minutes
Servings: 2
Total budget: 13$
Ingredients

- 2 tbsps. coconut oil
- 3 Chipotle chilies
- 2 tbsps. Adobo sauce
- 2 tsps. cumin
- 1 tsp. thyme, dried
- 1 tsp. salt
- 4 (5-oz.) pork chops, boneless
- ½ onion, chopped
- 2 bay leaves
- 1 cup chicken broth
- ½ (7-oz.) can tomatoes, fire-roasted and diced
- ⅓ cup cilantro, chopped

Directions

Melt the oil on Sauté in the Instant Pot. In a food processor, add salt, thyme, cumin, sauce, and chilies. Pulse to make a paste. Rub paste into the pork chops. Sear the chops in 5 minutes on each side. Add cilantro, tomatoes, broth, bay leaves, and onion to the Instant Pot. Close the lid and press Manual. Cook 15 min. on High. Do a natural release when done. Serve warm with cilantro garnish.

Nutrition
Calories: 375 kcal   **Total Fat:** 24.2 g   **Protein:** 31.3 g

Lunch Fish and Seafood Recipes

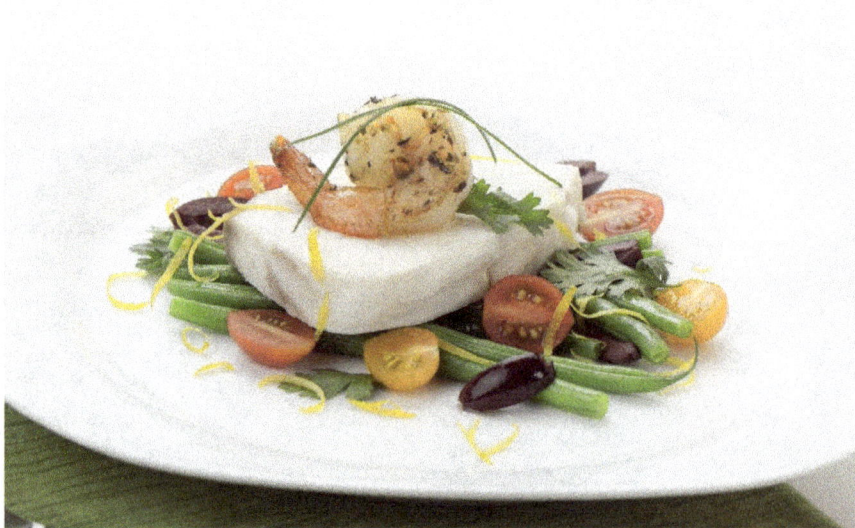

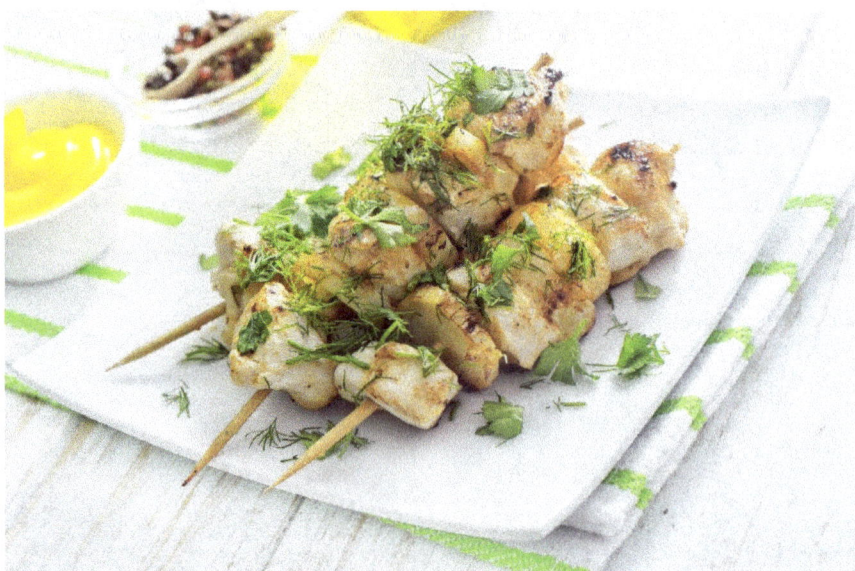

1. Tiger Prawn Risotto

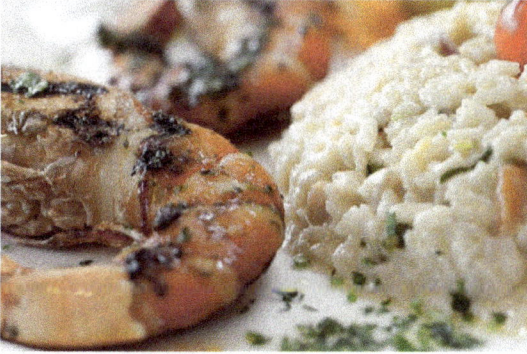

Preparation Time: 30 minutes
Cooking Time: 15 minutes
Servings: 2
Total budget: 15$
Ingredients

- Prawn Risotto
- 2 tbsps. coconut oil
- 5 tbsps. Shirataki rice
- 1 spring onion, sliced
- 4 tbsps. Parmesan cheese, grated
- 2 tbsps. baking soda
- 0.25 lbs. Tiger prawns, unpeeled, frozen
- 1 tbsp. low-sodium miso paste
- 1 tbsp. low sodium soy sauce
- 2 cups homemade fish stock
- 4 tbsps. cooking's sake
- 4 tbsps. Shirataki rice
- 8 tbsps. Shallot, minced
- 1 clove garlic, minced

- 2 tbsps. Butter, unsalted

Directions

To make the fish stock, add the ingredients to the Instant Pot cooker before sealing it and selecting the high-pressure setting for 5 mins. All the pressure to naturally release when the timer goes off. Set the stock aside. Set the Instant Pot to sauté before adding in the olive oil and butter and allowing it to heat up fully before adding in the shallots and garlic and allowing them to cook for about 3 mins. Add in the prawns and allow them to cook until they are mostly done. Remove them from the Instant Pot cooker and set them aside. Add to the rice and stir to coat evenly. Let it cook for two mins before adding in the miso paste and soy sauce and mixing well. Add in the cooking's sake to deglaze the pot. Let it boil for 60 seconds to ensure all the alcohol has evaporated. Add in the fish stock before sealing the lid of the cooker, choose the high pressure, and set the time for 5 mins. Peel the prawns while the risotto cooks. Once the timer goes off, select the instant pressure release option and remove the lid as soon as the pressure has normalized. If you prefer creamier risotto, then you will want to allow it to cook for an additional min. Toss in the onion and parmesan cheese and mix well prior to serving.

Nutrition

Calories: 221 kcal   **Total Fat:** 28 g   **Protein:** 12 g

2. Jambalaya

Preparation Time: 10 minutes
Cooking Time: 10 minutes
Servings: 2
Total budget: 15$

Ingredients

- 1 tsp. Worcestershire sauce
- 1 tsp. Creole seasoning
- ½ cup tomatoes, crushed
- 1-½ cup chicken stock
- 1-½ cup Shirataki rice
- 2 tbsps. garlic, minced
- 2 cups onion, diced fine
- 1 cup bell pepper, diced
- 0.25 lbs. prawns
- 0.25 lbs. chicken
- 2 tbsps. olive oil

Directions

Set the Instant Pot to sauté before coating the chicken using the creole seasoning and placing into the pot to brown completely. Once browned, remove it from the Instant Pot. Check the temperature with a meat thermometer, it should read close to 165°F. Add in the garlic, onion, and peppers and allow everything to sauté for about 5 mins or until the onion is brown. Add to the rice and stir to coat. Seal the lid of the cooker, choose the rice setting and leave the time at the default setting. Combine the remaining ingredients with the chicken and mix well. Once the timer goes off, select the instant pressure release option and remove the lid as soon as the pressure has normalized. Add in the remaining ingredients, reseal the lid, choose the high-pressure option and let everything cook for an additional 2 mins.

Nutrition
Calories: 321 kcal   **Total Fat:** 16.3 g   **Protein:** 21.1 g

3. Citrus Salmon

Preparation Time: 10 minutes
Cooking Time: 7 minutes
Servings: 2
Total budget: 15$

Ingredients

- 4 (4-oz.) salmon fillets
- 1 cup low-sodium chicken broth
- 1 tsp. ginger, fresh and minced
- 2 tsps. orange zest, fresh and grated finely
- 3 tbsps. orange juice, fresh
- 1 tbsp. olive oil
- ground black pepper, as required

Directions

In Instant Pot, add all ingredients and mix. Close lid and place the valve to "Seal" position. Press "Manual" and cook under "High Pressure" for about 7 mins. Press "Cancel" and allow a "Natural" release. Open the lid and serve the salmon fillets with the topping of cooking sauce.

Nutrition

Calories: 190 kcal **Total Fat:** 10.5 g

Dinner Vegetable Recipes

1. Steak Mushroom Sandwich

Preparation Time: 25 minutes
Cooking Time: 30 minutes
Servings: 2
Total budget: 14$

Ingredients

- 6 cloves garlic, crushed
- 1 cup balsamic vinegar
- 1 ½ lbs. steak skirt, strip or flank
- 1 spray olive oil
- ½ lb. Portobello mushrooms
- 4 whole-wheat hoagie rolls
- ½ tsp. kosher salt
- ¼ tsp. ground pepper

Directions

Mix vinegar and garlic in small-sized bowl and set it aside. Remove fat from steak. Heat large skillet to medium-high. Place steak in the skillet. Sear for two minutes. Turn steak and cook for 2 minutes more, till done as you desire. Remove steak from skillet. Set it aside. Spray oil in the skillet to coat. Add mushrooms. Cook for 5 minutes and turn them once. Remove to cutting board.

Add vinegar and garlic mixture to skillet. Boil for 3 to 4 mins, till it reduces by ½. Divide sauce among 4 individual bowls. Set them aside. Slice rolls open. Mist both sides with spray of oil. Toast rolls in toaster oven for a min. Slice steak mushrooms in thin strips. Arrange 5 oz. steak ¾ cup mushrooms on bottom halves of rolls. Top that with

kosher salt and ground pepper. Cover sandwiches with top halves. Cut sandwiches in ½. Serve with dipping sauce.
Nutrition: Calories: 485 kcal   **Total Fat:** 13 g **Protein:** 45 g

2. Sweet Potatoes with Roast Chicken
Preparation Time: 50 minutes
Cooking Time: 60 minutes
Servings: 2
Total budget: 9$
Ingredients
- 2 tbsps. Dijon mustard, or whole grain
- 2 tbsps. thyme, fresh and chopped
- 2 tbsps. olive oil
- ½ tsp. kosher salt
- ½ tsp. ground pepper
- 1 ½ to 2 lbs. chicken thighs, de-skinned, bone-in
- 2 medium sweet potatoes, peeled, 1-inch cut
- 1 large red onion, 1 x 1-inch wedge cut

Directions

Position the rack in lower ⅓ of your oven. Preheat it to 450°F. Place large cookie sheet with rim in the oven and preheat it. Combine 1 tbsp. oil, thyme, mustard, and ¼ tsp. each kosher salt and ground pepper in small mixing bowl. Evenly spread mixture on the chicken. Toss onions and sweet potatoes in medium bowl with last 1 tbsp. oil and remainder of kosher salt and ground pepper. Remove cookie sheet carefully from oven. Spread veggies on it. Then place chicken on the top. Return cookie sheet to oven. Roast and stir veggies halfway through cooking time, till vegetables become tender and start browning. Internal meat temperature should be 165°F and no pink should remain, 30–35 mins. Remove from oven and serve.

Nutrition: Calories: 406 kcal   **Total Fat:** 16.9 g
Protein: 27 g

3. BBQ Broccoli Ranch Wraps

Preparation Time: 15 minutes
Cooking Time: 20 minutes
Servings: 2
Total budget: 8$
Ingredients

- 2 tbsps. ranch dressing, reduced-fat, bottled
- 1 tbsp. mayonnaise dressing, light
- 2 cups broccoli, pre-packaged, shredded
- 4 x 8-inches whole-grain tortilla flours
- 2 tbsps. BBQ sauce, bottled
- 8 oz. turkey or chicken breast, shredded and cooked

Directions

In medium mixing bowl, combine the ranch dressing with mayo dressing. Add and stir in the broccoli shreds. Spread the tortillas with bottled BBQ sauce and top them with chicken. Add broccoli mixture atop chicken. Roll tortillas up and serve.

Nutrition

Calories: 276 kcal   **Total Fat:** 6.9 g   **Protein:** 21.9 g

Dinner Meat Recipes

1. Pork with Mushrooms and Cucumbers

Preparation Time: 15 minutes
Cooking Time: 25 minutes
Servings: 2
Total budget: 7$
Ingredients

- 2 tbsps. olive oil
- ½ tsp. oregano, dried
- 4 pork chops
- 2 garlic cloves, minced
- Juice of 1 lime
- ¼ cup cilantro, chopped
- A pinch sea salt and black pepper
- 1 cup white mushrooms, halved
- 2 tbsps. balsamic vinegar

Directions

Heat the pan with the oil with a medium heat, add the pork chops and brown for 2 mins on each side. Add rest of the ingredients, toss, cook over medium heat for 20 mins, divide between plates.

Nutrition

Calories: 220 kcal   **Total Fat:** 6 g   **Protein:** 20 g   **Fiber** 8 g

2. Chicken Chopstick

Preparation Time: 15 minutes
Cooking Time: 25 minutes
Servings: 2
Total budget: 8$
Ingredients

- ¼ cup onion, diced and chopped
- 1 pack chow Mein noodles, cooked
- ground pepper, fresh
- 2 cans cream mushroom soup
- 1 ¼ cup celery, sliced
- 1 cup cashew nuts
- 2 cups chicken, cubed and cooked
- ½ cup water

Directions

Preheat the oven to 375°F. In a pot suitable for the oven, pour in both cans of cream of mushroom soup and water. Mix until combined. Add the cooked cubed chicken, onion, celery, pepper, cashew nuts to the soup. Stir until combined. Add half the noodles to the mixture, stir until coated.

Top the casserole with the rest of the noodles. Place the pot in the oven. Bake for 25 mins.

Nutrition
Calories: 201 kcal   **Total Fat:** 17 g   **Protein:** 13 g

3. Balsamic Roast Chicken

Preparation Time: 25 minutes
Cooking Time: 50 minutes
Servings: 2
Total budget: 10$
Ingredients

- 1 tbsp. fresh rosemary, minced
- 1 garlic clove, minced
- Black pepper
- 1 tbsp. olive oil
- 1 tsp. brown sugar
- 6 rosemary sprigs
- 1 whole chicken
- ½ cup balsamic vinegar

Directions

Combine garlic, minced rosemary, black pepper, and the olive oil. Rub the chicken with the herbal olive oil mixture. Put 3 rosemary sprigs into the chicken cavity. Place the chicken into a roasting pan and roast at 400°F for about 1 hr. 30 mins. When the chicken is golden, and the juices run clear, transfer to a serving dish. In a saucepan, dissolve the sugar in balsamic vinegar overheat. Do not boil. Carve the chicken and top with vinegar mixture.

Nutrition

Calories: 587 kcal   **Total Fat:** 37.8 g   **Protein:** 54.1 g

4. Steak & Mushrooms

Preparation Time: 5 minutes
Cooking Time: 15 minutes
Servings: 2
Total budget: 15$

Ingredients

- 2 tbsps. olive oil
- 8 oz. mushrooms, sliced
- ½ tsp. garlic powder
- 1 lb. steak, sliced into cubes
- 1 tsp. Worcestershire sauce
- Pepper to taste

Directions

Preheat air fryer to 400°F. Combine all ingredients in a bowl. Transfer to the air fryer basket. Cook for 15 mins, shaking the basket twice.

Nutrition

Calories: 927 kcal   **Total Fat:** 37.6 g   **Carbs:** 88.7 g
Protein: 74.5 g

Dinner Fish and Seafood

1. Salmon & Shrimp Stew
Preparation Time: 20 minutes
Cooking Time: 21 minutes
Servings: 2
Total budget: 15$
Ingredients

- 2 tbsps. olive oil
- ½ cup onion, chopped finely
- 2 garlic cloves, minced
- 1 Serrano pepper, chopped
- 1 tsp. paprika, smoked
- 4 cups tomatoes, fresh and chopped
- 4 cups low-sodium chicken broth
- 1-lb. salmon fillets, cubed
- 1-lb. shrimp, peeled and deveined
- 2 tbsps. lime juice, fresh
- ¼ cup basil, fresh and chopped
- ¼ cup parsley, fresh and chopped
- Ground black pepper, as required
- 2 scallions, chopped

Directions

In a large soup pan, melt coconut oil over medium-high heat and sauté the onion for about 5–6 mins. Add the garlic, Serrano pepper, and smoked paprika, and sauté for about 1 minute. Add the tomatoes and broth and bring to a gentle simmer over medium heat. Simmer for about 5 mins. Add the salmon and simmer for about 3–4 mins. Stir in the remaining seafood and cook for about 4–5 mins. Stir in the lemon juice, basil, parsley, sea salt, and black pepper and remove from heat. Serve it hot with the garnishing of scallion.

Nutrition

Calories: 271 kcal **Total Fat:** 11 g **Protein:** 34.7 g

2. Salmon Curry
Preparation Time: 15 minutes
Cooking Time: 30 minutes
Servings: 2
Total budget: 11$
Ingredients
- (4-oz.) salmon fillets
- 1 tsp. ground turmeric, divided
- Salt, as required
- 3 tbsps. olive oil, divided
- 1 yellow onion, chopped finely
- 1 tsp. garlic paste
- 1 tsp. ginger paste, fresh
- 3–4 green chilies, halved
- 1 tsp. red chili powder
- ½ tsp. ground cumin
- ½ tsp. ground cinnamon
- ¾ cup plain Greek yogurt, fat-free, whipped
- ¾ cup water, filtered
- 3 tbsps. cilantro, fresh and chopped

Directions
Season each salmon fillet with ½ tsp. turmeric and salt. In the large skillet, melt 1 tbsp. butter over medium heat and cook the salmon fillets for about 2 mins per side. Transfer the salmon onto a plate. In the same skillet, melt the remaining butter over medium heat and sauté the onion for

about 4–5 mins. Add the garlic paste, ginger paste, green chilies, remaining turmeric, and spices and sauté for about 1 min. Now, reduce the heat to medium-low. Slowly, add the yogurt and water, stirring continuously until smooth. Cover the skillet and simmer for about 10–15 mins or until desired doneness of the sauce. Carefully, add the salmon fillets and simmer for about 5 mins. Serve it hot with cilantro.

Nutrition

Calories: 242 kcal   **Total Fat:** 14.3 g   **Protein:** 25.4 g

3. Salmon with Bell Peppers
Preparation Time: 15 minutes
Cooking Time: 20 minutes
Servings: 2
Total budget: 11$
Ingredients

- 6 (3-oz.) salmon fillets
- Pinch salt
- Ground black pepper, as required
- 1 yellow bell pepper, seeded and cubed
- 1 red bell pepper, seeded and cubed
- 4 plum tomatoes, cubed
- 1 small onion, sliced thinly
- ½ cup parsley, fresh and chopped
- ¼ cup olive oil
- 2 tbsps. lemon juice, fresh

Directions

Preheat the oven to 400°F. Season each of the salmon fillets with salt and black pepper lightly. In a bowl, mix the bell peppers, tomato, and onion. Arrange 6 foil pieces onto a smooth surface. Place 1 salmon fillet over each foil paper and sprinkle with salt and black pepper. Place veggie mixture over each fillet evenly and top with parsley and capers evenly. Drizzle with oil and lemon juice.

Fold each foil around salmon mixture to seal it. Arrange the foil packets onto a large baking sheet in a single layer. Bake for about 20 mins.

Nutrition
Calories: 220 kcal   **Total Fat:** 14 g   **Protein:** 17.9 g

4. Shrimp Salad
Preparation Time: 20 minutes
Cooking Time: 4 minutes
Servings: 2
Total budget: 13$
Ingredients
For Salad:

- 1-lb. shrimp, peeled and deveined
- Salt and ground black pepper, as required
- 1 tsp. olive oil
- 1½ cups carrots, peeled and julienned
- 1½ cups red cabbage, shredded
- 1½ cup cucumber, julienned
- 5 cups baby arugula, fresh
- ¼ cup basil, fresh and chopped
- ¼ cup cilantro, fresh and chopped
- 4 cups lettuce, torn
- ¼ cup almonds, chopped

For Dressing:

- 2 tbsps. natural almond butter
- 1 garlic clove, crushed
- 1 tbsp. cilantro, fresh and chopped
- 1 tbsp. lime juice, fresh
- 1 tbsp. applesauce, unsweetened
- 2 tsps. balsamic vinegar
- ½ tsp. cayenne pepper
- Salt, as required
- 1 tbsp. water

- ⅓ cup olive oil

Directions

Slowly, add the oil, beating continuously until smooth.

For salad: In a bowl, add shrimp, salt, black pepper, and oil and toss to coat well.

Heat the skillet over medium-high heat and cook the shrimp for about 2 mins per side. Remove from the heat and set aside to cool. In a large bowl, add the shrimp, vegetables and mix well.

For dressing: In a bowl, add all ingredients except oil and beat until well combined. Place the dressing over shrimp mixture and gently, toss to coat well.

Nutrition: Calories: 274 kcal   **Total Fat:** 17.7 g **Protein:** 20.5 g

Appetizers and Side Dishes

1. Fish with Fresh Tomato - Basil Sauce

Preparation Time: 10 minutes

Cooking Time: 15 minutes

Serving: 2

Total budget: 8$

Ingredients

- 2 (4-oz.) tilapia fillets
- 1 tbsp. fresh basil, chopped
- ⅛ tsp. salt
- A pinch red pepper, crushed
- 1 cup cherry tomatoes, chopped
- 2 tsps. extra virgin olive oil

Directions

Preheat oven to 400°F. Arrange rinsed and patted dry fish fillets on foil (coat a foil baking sheet with cooking spray). Sprinkle tilapia fillets with salt and red pepper. Bake 12–15 mins. Meanwhile, mix leftover ingredients in a saucepan. Cook over medium-high heat until tomatoes are tender. Top fish fillets properly with tomato mixture.

Nutrition

Calories: 130 kcal   **Carbs:** 1 g   **Protein:** 30 g

2. Mashed Pumpkin

Preparation Time: 9 minutes
Cooking Time: 15 minutes
Servings: 2
Total budget: 7$

Ingredients

- 2 cups pumpkin, chopped
- ½ cup water
- 2 tbsps. powdered sweetener of choice, sugar-free
- 1 tbsp. cinnamon

Directions

Place the pumpkin and water in your Instant Pot. Seal and cook on Stew 15 mins. Remove and mash with the sweetener and cinnamon.

Nutrition

Calories: 12 kcal   **Carbs:** 3 g   **Sugar:** 1 g

3. Parmesan-Topped Acorn Squash

Preparation Time: 8 minutes
Cooking Time: 20 minutes
Servings: 2
Total budget: 10$
Ingredients

- 1 corn squash (about 1 lb.)
- 1 tbsp. extra-virgin olive oil
- 1 tsp. sage leaves, dried and crumbled
- ¼ tsp. nutmeg, freshly grated
- ⅛ tsp. kosher salt
- ⅛ tsp. freshly ground black pepper
- 2 tbsps. Parmesan cheese, freshly grated

Directions

Chop acorn squash in half lengthwise and remove the seeds. Cut each half in half for a total of 4 wedges. Snap off the stem if it is easy to do. In a small bowl, combine the olive oil, sage, nutmeg, salt, and pepper. Brush the cut sides of the squash with the olive oil mixture. Fill 1 cup water into the electric pressure cooker and insert a wire rack or trivet. Place the squash on the trivet in a single layer, skin-side down. Set the lid of the pressure cooker on sealing. Cook on high pressure for 20 mins. Once done, press Cancel and quick release the pressure. Once the pin drops, open it. Carefully remove the squash from the pot, sprinkle with the Parmesan, and serve.

Nutrition
Calories: 85 kcal   **Carbs:** 12 g   **Fiber:** 2 g

4. Quinoa Tabbouleh
Preparation Time: 8 minutes
Cooking Time: 16 minutes
Servings: 2
Total budget: 10$
Ingredients

- 1 cup quinoa, rinsed
- 1 large English cucumber
- 2 scallions, sliced
- 2 cups cherry tomatoes, halved
- ⅔ cup parsley, chopped
- ½ cup mint, chopped
- ½ tsp. garlic, minced
- ½ tsp. salt
- ½ tsp. ground black pepper
- 2 tbsps. lemon juice
- ½ cup olive oil

Directions

Plugin instant pot, insert the inner pot, add quinoa, then pour in water and stir until mixed. Close instant pot with its lid and turn the pressure knob to seal the pot. Select 'manual' button, then set the 'timer' to 1 minute and cook in high pressure, it may take 7 mins. Once the timer stops, select 'cancel' button and do natural pressure release for 10 mins, and then do quick pressure release until pressure nob drops down. Open the instant pot, fluff quinoa with a fork, then spoon it on a rimmed baking sheet, spread quinoa evenly and let cool. Meanwhile, place lime juice in a small bowl, add garlic, and stir until just mixed. Then add salt, black pepper, and olive oil and whisk until combined. Transfer cooled quinoa to a large bowl, add remaining ingredients, then drizzle generously with the prepared lime juice mixture and toss until evenly coated. Taste quinoa to adjust seasoning.

Nutrition

Calories: 283 kcal **Carbs:** 30.6 g Fiber 3.4 g

5. Wild Rice Salad with Cranberries and Almonds
Preparation Time: 6 minutes
Cooking Time: 25 minutes
Servings: 2
Total budget: 9$
Ingredients
For the rice:

- 2 cups wild rice blend, rinsed
- 1 tsp. kosher salt
- 2½ cups Vegetable Broth

For the dressing:

- ¼ cup extra-virgin olive oil
- ¼ cup white wine vinegar
- 1½ tsps. orange zest, grated
- Juice of 1 medium orange (about ¼ cup)
- 1 tsp. honey or pure maple syrup

For the salad:

- ¾ cup cranberries, unsweetened, dried
- ½ cup almonds, sliced and toasted
- freshly ground black pepper

Directions
To make the rice: In the electric pressure cooker, combine the rice, salt, and broth. Close and lock the lid. Set the valve to sealing. Cook on high pressure for 25 mins. When the cooking is complete, hit Cancel and allow the pressure to release naturally for 1minutes, then quick release any remaining pressure. Once the pin drops, unlock and remove the lid. Let the rice cool briefly, then fluff it with a fork. **To make the dressing:** While the rice cooks, make

the dressing: In a small jar with a screw-top lid, combine the olive oil, vinegar, zest, juice, and honey. (If you do not have a jar, whisk the ingredients together in a small bowl.) Shake to combine. **To make the salad:** Mix rice, cranberries, and almonds. Add the dressing and season with pepper. Serve warm or refrigerate.

Nutrition

Calories: 126 kcal   **Carbs:** 18 g   **Fiber:** 2 g

6. Low Fat Toasties
Preparation Time: 8 minutes
Cooking Time: 25 minutes
Servings: 2
Total budget: 6$
Ingredients

- 1 lb. roasting potatoes
- 1 garlic clove
- 1 cup vegetable stock
- 2 tbsps. olive oil

Directions

Position potatoes in the steamer basket and add the stock into the Instant Pot. Steam the potatoes in your Instant Pot for 15 mins. Depressurize and pour away the remaining stock. Set to sauté and add the oil, garlic, and potatoes. Cook until brown.

Nutrition
Calories: 201 kcal   **Total Fat:** 6 g   **Carbs:** 3 g

7. Roasted Parsnips
Preparation Time: 9 minutes
Cooking Time: 25 minutes
Servings: 2
Total budget: 8$
Ingredients

-
- 1 lb. parsnips
- 1 cup vegetable stock
- 2 tbsps. herbs
- 2 tbsps. olive oil

Directions

Put the parsnips in the steamer basket and add the stock into the Instant Pot. Steam the parsnips in your Instant Pot for 15 mins. Depressurize and pour away the remaining stock. Set to sauté and add the oil, herbs, and parsnips. Cook until golden and crisp.

Nutrition
Calories: 130 kcal   **Carbs:** 14 g   **Protein:** 4 g

8. Lower Carb Hummus

Preparation Time: 9 minutes
Cooking Time: 60 minutes
Servings: 2
Total budget: 8$

Ingredients

- ½ cup dry chickpeas
- 1 cup vegetable stock
- 1 cup pumpkin puree
- 2 tbsps. paprika, smoked
- salt and pepper to taste

Directions

Soak the chickpeas overnight. Place the chickpeas and stock in the Instant Pot. Cook on Beans 60 mins. Depressurize naturally. Blend the chickpeas with the remaining ingredients.

Nutrition

Calories: 135 kcal   **Total Fat:** 3 g   **Carbs:** 18 g

9. Chili Sin Carne

Preparation Time: 30 minutes
Cooking Time: 35 minutes
Servings: 2
Total budget: 9$
Ingredients

- 3 cups mixed beans, cooked
- 2 cups tomatoes, chopped
- 2 squares very dark chocolate
- 1tbsp red chili flakes + 1tbsp yeast extract

Directions

Mix all the ingredients in your Instant Pot. Cook on Beans for 35 mins. Release the pressure.

Nutrition

Calories: 200 kcal   **Total Fat:** 3 g   **Carbs:** 20 g   Sugar 5g   **Protein:** 36 g

Snack and Dessert

1. Fruit Kebab
Preparation Time: 10 minutes
Cooking Time: 30 minutes
Ingredients
Servings: 2
Total budget: 8$

- 3 apples
- ¼ cup orange juice
- 1 ½ lb. watermelon
- ¾ cup blueberries

Directions

Use a star-shaped cookie cutter to cut out stars from the apple and watermelon. Soak the apple stars in orange juice. Thread the apple stars, watermelon stars, and blueberries into skewers. Refrigerate for 30 mins before serving.

Nutrition
Calories: 52 kcal   **Total Fat:** 0 g   **Protein:** 1 g

2. Cheese Berry Fat Bomb

Preparation Time: 10 minutes

Cooking Time: 30 minutes

Servings: 2

Total budget: 6$

Ingredients

- 1 cup berries, fresh and washed
- ½ cup coconut oil
- 1 ½ cup cream cheese, softened
- 1 tbsp. vanilla
- 2 tbsps. Swerve

Directions

Add all ingredients to the blender and blend until smooth and combined. Spoon mixture into small candy molds and refrigerate until set. Serve and enjoy!

Nutrition

Calories: 175 kcal **Total Fat:** 17 g **Protein:** 2.1 g

3. Tamari Toasted Almonds

Preparation Time: 10 minutes
Cooking Time: 30 minutes
Servings: 2
Total budget: 7$

Ingredients

- ½ cup raw almonds, or sunflower seeds
- 2 tsps. tamari, or soy sauce
- 1 tsp. sesame oil, toasted

Directions

Preparing the ingredients.Heat a dry skillet to medium-high heat, then add the almonds, stirring frequently to keep them from burning. Once the almonds are toasted (7–8 mins for almonds, or 34 mins for sunflower seeds), pour the tamari and sesame oil into the hot skillet and stir to coat. You can turn off the heat, and as the almonds cool, the tamari mixture will stick and dry on to the nuts.

Nutrition: Calories: 89 kcal **Total Fat:** 8 g **Protein:** 4 g

4. Choco Peppermint Cake
Preparation Time: 10 minutes
Cooking Time: 30 minutes
Servings: 2
Total budget: 5$
Ingredients
- Cooking spray
- ⅓ cup oil
- 15 oz. package chocolate cake mix
- 3 eggs, beaten
- 1 cup water
- ¼ tsp. peppermint extract

Directions
Spray slow cooker with oil. Mix all the ingredients in a bowl. Use an electric mixer on medium speed setting to mix ingredients for 2 mins. Pour mixture into the slow cooker. Cover the pot and cook on low for 3 hours. Let cool before slicing and serving.

Nutrition: Calories: 185 kcal   **Total Fat:** 7.4 g   **Protein:** 3.8 g

5. Frozen Lemon & Blueberry
Preparation Time: 10 minutes
Cooking Time: 30 minutes
Total budget: 5$
Servings: 2
Ingredients

- 6 cups blueberries, fresh
- 8 sprigs thyme, fresh
- ¾ cup light brown sugar
- 1 tsp. lemon zest
- ¼ cup lemon juice
- 2 cups water

Directions

Add blueberries, thyme, and sugar in a pan over medium heat. Cook for 6 to 8 minutes. Transfer mixture to a blender. Remove thyme sprigs. Stir in the remaining ingredients. Pulse until smooth. Strain mixture and freeze for 1 hour.

Nutrition: Calories: 78 kcal   **Total Fat:** 0 g   **Protein:** 3 g

6. Pumpkin & Banana Ice Cream

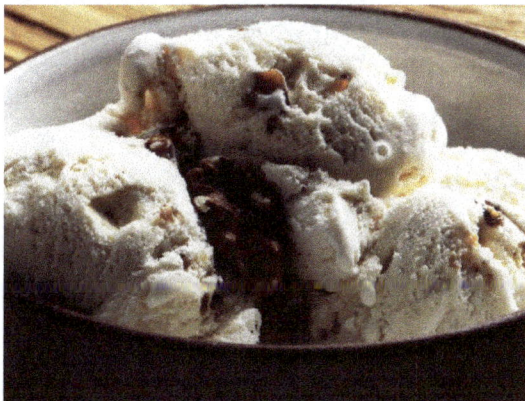

Preparation Time: 10 minutes
Cooking Time: 30 minutes
Servings: 2
Total budget: 8$
Ingredients

- 15 oz. pumpkin puree
- 4 bananas, sliced and frozen
- 1 tsp. pumpkin pie spice
- Pecans, chopped

Directions

Add pumpkin puree, bananas, and pumpkin pie spice in a food processor. Pulse until smooth. Chill in the refrigerator. Garnish with pecans.

Nutrition

Calories: 71 kcal   **Total Fat:** 0.4 g   **Protein:** 1.2 g

7. Coconut Chia Pudding

Preparation Time: 10 minutes
Cooking Time: 0 minutes

Servings: 2
Total budget: 7$
Ingredients

- 2 ¼ cup coconut milk, canned
- 1 tsp. vanilla extract
- A pinch salt
- ½ cup chia seeds

Directions

Combine the coconut milk, vanilla, and salt in a bowl. Stir well and sweeten with stevia to taste.

Whisk in the chia seeds and chill overnight. Spoon into bowls and serve with chopped nuts or fruit.

Nutrition

Calories: 300 kcal   **Total Fat:** 27.5 g   **Protein:** 6 g

8. Strawberries in Honey Yogurt Dip
Preparation Time: 10 minutes
Cooking Time: 0 minutes
Servings: 2
Total budget: 7$
Ingredients

- 1 cup plain yogurt, low-fat
- 1 tbsp. orange juice
- 1 tsp. honey
- Ground cinnamon
- ¼ strawberries, fresh (remove stems)

Directions

Combine first four ingredients to make a sauce. Pour over strawberries and serve.

Nutrition
Calories: 88 kcal   **Total Fat:** 1 g   **Protein:** 4 g

9. Tiramisu Shots
Preparation Time: 5 minutes
Cooking Time: 10 minutes
Servings: 2
Total budget: 5$
Ingredients

- 1 pack silken tofu
- 1 oz. dark chocolate, finely chopped
- ¼ cup sugar substitute
- 1 tsp. lemon juice
- ¼ cup espresso, brewed
- Pinch salt
- 24 slices angel food cake
- Cocoa powder, unsweetened

Directions

Add tofu, chocolate, sugar substitute, lemon juice, espresso, and salt in a food processor. Pulse until smooth. Add angel food cake pieces into shot glasses. Drizzle with the cocoa powder. Pour the tofu mixture on top. Top with the remaining angel food cake pieces. Chill for 30 mins and serve.

Nutrition
Calories: 75 kcal   **Protein:** 2.9 g

CPSIA information can be obtained
at www.ICGtesting.com
Printed in the USA
BVHW091055090621
609091BV00009B/1019